CIALIS

A Comprehensive Guide to Cialis and Reclaiming Your Intimate Well-being

Dr. Rose Grey

TABLE OF CONTENTS

CHAPTER 1
INTRODUCTION

In the realm of men's health, the topic of erectile dysfunction (ED) is both delicate and prevalent. Millions of men around the world face the challenges associated with ED, impacting not only their physical well-being but also their emotional and psychological health. Cialis, featuring the active ingredient Tadalafil, stands as a beacon of hope for those navigating the complexities of this condition.

This comprehensive guide aims to shed light on the multifaceted aspects of Cialis, providing readers with a thorough understanding of its mechanisms, applications, and the impact it can have on one's life. From the historical roots of ED to the cutting-edge science behind Cialis, this book endeavors to demystify the subject, fostering a sense of empowerment and knowledge for those seeking solutions.

Historical Background

To appreciate the present, it is crucial to understand the past. The historical exploration in this book delves into the evolution of ED treatments and the development of Cialis. From the early discoveries that paved the way for advancements in men's health to the specific milestones leading to the creation of Cialis, this section sets the stage for a comprehensive journey through time.

Purpose and Scope of the Book

Why Cialis? What sets it apart from other ED medications? The purpose of this guide is not only to answer these questions but also to equip readers with the knowledge needed to make informed decisions about their health. From the intricacies of Tadalafil's mechanism of action to practical tips for incorporating Cialis into daily life, this book aims to be a valuable resource for individuals, partners, and healthcare professionals alike.

Embark on this exploration of Cialis, where science meets lived experiences, and the pursuit of well-being takes center stage. Whether you are a curious reader, someone dealing with ED, or a healthcare professional seeking to enhance patient care, this guide invites you to navigate the world of Cialis with curiosity, confidence, and the assurance that you are not alone in your journey toward optimal health and vitality.

CHAPTER 2
UNDERSTANDING ERECTILE DYSFUNCTION

Erectile Dysfunction (ED) is a pervasive and often misunderstood condition that affects men of various ages. This section aims to unravel the complexities of ED, offering insights into its definition, causes, and the profound impact it can have on individuals and their relationships.

Definition and Causes

Defining Erectile Dysfunction: Explore a comprehensive definition of ED, distinguishing between occasional difficulties and persistent challenges.

Physical Factors: Investigate the role of physical health in ED, covering aspects such as cardiovascular health, hormonal imbalances, and neurological conditions.

Psychological Factors: Delve into the intricate connection between the mind and erectile function, discussing stress, anxiety, depression, and other psychological contributors.

Medical Conditions

Cardiovascular Diseases: Examine the strong correlation between heart health and erectile function, understanding how conditions like hypertension and atherosclerosis can contribute to ED.

Endocrine Disorders: Explore the impact of hormonal imbalances, including conditions such as diabetes and low testosterone levels, on erectile function.

Neurological Disorders: Investigate the role of the nervous system in ED, exploring conditions like multiple sclerosis and Parkinson's disease.

Lifestyle Factors

Smoking and Alcohol: Assess the impact of smoking and excessive alcohol consumption on erectile function, highlighting lifestyle modifications for improvement.

Diet and Exercise: Understand the significance of a healthy lifestyle, incorporating balanced nutrition and regular physical activity as essential components of ED prevention and management.

The Psychological Toll of ED

Impact on Mental Health: Discuss the emotional consequences of living with ED, addressing self-esteem issues, relationship strains, and the importance of open communication.

Seeking Professional Help: Encourage a proactive approach to seeking medical and psychological assistance, emphasizing the importance of collaboration between individuals and healthcare providers.

This section serves as a foundational exploration, setting the stage for the subsequent chapters that delve into the science behind Cialis and its role in addressing the challenges posed by ED. By understanding the intricacies of this condition, readers can approach the journey toward solutions with informed perspectives and a renewed sense of agency.

CHAPTER 3
THE SCIENCE BEHIND CIALIS

Cialis, featuring the active ingredient Tadalafil, stands at the forefront of medical advancements in the treatment of erectile dysfunction (ED). This section aims to unravel the scientific intricacies that make Cialis a unique and effective solution for individuals facing the challenges of ED.

Tadalafil: The Active Ingredient

Chemical Composition: Explore the chemical structure of Tadalafil, delving into its pharmacological properties and how it sets itself apart from other phosphodiesterase type 5 (PDE5) inhibitors.

Mechanism of Action: Uncover the precise mechanisms through which Tadalafil operates in the body, elucidating how it facilitates increased blood flow to the penis and the promotion of erectile function.

Duration of Action: Understand the prolonged duration of Cialis's effects, differentiating it from other ED medications and offering a unique advantage for individuals seeking spontaneity in their intimate relationships.

How Cialis Differs from Other ED Medications

Comparative Analysis: Conduct a comparative analysis of Cialis against other commonly prescribed ED medications, highlighting the distinct features that make Cialis a preferred choice for certain individuals.

Onset of Action: Discuss the relatively rapid onset of action of Cialis, providing insights into how this characteristic contributes to its versatility as both a daily and as-needed medication.

Interaction with Food and Alcohol: Examine how the absorption of Tadalafil is influenced by food and alcohol, offering practical advice for individuals looking to optimize the effectiveness of Cialis.

Safety and Side Effects

Safety Profile: Evaluate the safety profile of Cialis, emphasizing its approval by regulatory authorities and the importance of obtaining a prescription for proper use.

Common Side Effects: Address the potential side effects associated with Cialis, offering guidance on recognizing and managing these effects to ensure a positive and safe experience.

Precautions and Contraindications: Highlight specific precautions and contraindications associated with Cialis, emphasizing the importance of consulting with a healthcare professional before use.

Patient Experience

Real-time Vasodilation: Explain the impact of Tadalafil on the relaxation of smooth muscle tissue, elucidating how this process contributes to increased blood flow and improved erectile function.

By delving into the science behind Cialis, readers can gain a profound understanding of how this medication operates on a physiological level, empowering them to make informed decisions about its use in addressing the complexities of erectile dysfunction.

CHAPTER 4
EXPLORING CIALIS VARIANTS

Cialis, with its active ingredient Tadalafil, offers a range of options to address the diverse needs and preferences of individuals dealing with erectile dysfunction (ED). This section navigates through the different variants of Cialis, providing insights into their unique features, applications, and considerations.

Cialis Daily

Introduction to Cialis Daily: Understand the concept of daily-use Cialis, exploring how it differs from the as-needed version and the advantages it offers for individuals seeking continuous ED support.

Low-Dose Formulation: Examine the lower daily dosage of Tadalafil in Cialis Daily, discussing how this steady, low-dose approach can provide ongoing benefits without the need for planning ahead.

Spontaneity and Daily Use: Highlight the increased spontaneity associated with Cialis Daily, allowing users to engage in sexual activity without the constraints of timing their medication.

Cialis as Needed

Flexibility of Use: Explore the on-demand nature of Cialis as needed, providing insights into how this variant allows users to take the medication when anticipation and timing are crucial.

Higher Dosage Options: Discuss the higher dosage options available for as-needed Cialis, offering flexibility for individuals with varying needs and responses.

Timing Considerations: Provide guidance on the optimal timing for taking Cialis as needed, ensuring users can maximize the effectiveness of the medication during intimate moments.

Generic Cialis: What You Need to Know

Introduction to Generic Cialis: Understand the emergence of generic versions of Cialis, exploring how they compare to the brand-name medication in terms of efficacy, safety, and cost.

Regulatory Approval: Discuss the regulatory processes governing generic medications, assuring readers of the standards these alternatives must meet for approval.

Cost Considerations: Examine the cost-effectiveness of generic Cialis, offering insights into how these alternatives may provide affordable options for individuals seeking ED treatment.

Tailoring Cialis to Individual Needs

Consulting with Healthcare Professionals: Emphasize the importance of consulting with healthcare professionals to determine the most suitable Cialis variant based on individual health conditions, preferences, and lifestyle.

Combining Variants: Discuss the potential for combining different Cialis variants, exploring scenarios where a combination approach may be beneficial for certain individuals.

Considering Partner Perspectives: Address the impact of Cialis variants on intimate relationships, encouraging open communication and collaboration between individuals and their partners.

By exploring the diverse array of Cialis variants, readers can gain a nuanced understanding of how these options cater to different lifestyles and preferences, allowing individuals to tailor their ED treatment to best suit their unique needs.

CHAPTER 5
LIFESTYLE AND CIALIS

The integration of Cialis, with its active ingredient Tadalafil, into one's lifestyle goes beyond the mere administration of a medication. This section explores the symbiotic relationship between lifestyle choices and the effectiveness of Cialis in addressing erectile dysfunction (ED). By embracing a holistic approach, individuals can optimize the benefits of Cialis while cultivating a healthier overall lifestyle.

Integrating Cialis into Daily Life

Incorporating Cialis into Routine: Provide practical advice on seamlessly integrating Cialis into daily life, emphasizing the importance of consistency for those using the daily variant.

Planning for Spontaneity: Discuss strategies for incorporating as-needed Cialis into a lifestyle that values spontaneity, ensuring individuals can enjoy the flexibility this variant offers.

Communication with Partners: Encourage open communication between individuals and their partners about the incorporation of Cialis into the relationship, fostering understanding and shared expectations.

Tips for a Healthy Lifestyle

Nutrition and Exercise: Highlight the role of a balanced diet and regular physical activity in promoting overall health, addressing how these lifestyle factors contribute to improved vascular function—a key aspect of erectile health.

Stress Management: Explore stress-reduction techniques, recognizing the impact of stress on ED and providing practical suggestions for managing stress in daily life.

Adequate Sleep: Emphasize the importance of quality sleep in supporting overall well-being, including its positive effects on hormonal balance and mental health.

Combining Cialis with Other Treatments

Holistic Approach to ED: Discuss the potential benefits of combining Cialis with other ED treatments, such as psychotherapy, lifestyle modifications, or alternative therapies, providing a comprehensive approach to addressing the multifaceted nature of ED.

Smoking Cessation and Moderation of Alcohol: Address the detrimental effects of smoking and excessive alcohol consumption on erectile function, offering guidance on lifestyle changes to complement the use of Cialis.

Regular Health Check-ups: Stress the importance of regular health check-ups and consultations with healthcare professionals, ensuring that any underlying health issues contributing to ED are promptly addressed.

Personalizing the Cialis Experience

Dosage Adjustments: Discuss considerations for adjusting Cialis dosage based on individual responses and needs, encouraging individuals to work closely with healthcare professionals to optimize their treatment plan.

Understanding Individual Triggers: Explore the role of individual triggers for ED, empowering individuals to identify and address lifestyle factors that may contribute to their specific condition.

Sustainable Changes: Advocate for sustainable lifestyle changes, emphasizing the long-term benefits of adopting healthy habits that extend beyond the immediate management of ED.

By intertwining lifestyle adjustments with the use of Cialis, individuals can embark on a journey that not only addresses the challenges of erectile dysfunction but also fosters a holistic approach to well-being. This section aims to empower readers to take charge of their health, recognizing that the synergy of lifestyle choices and medical interventions contributes to a more comprehensive and enduring solution to ED.

CHAPTER 6
CONCLUSION

As we reach the culmination of this exploration into the world of Cialis, it becomes evident that the journey from understanding erectile dysfunction to embracing Cialis as a solution is multifaceted and deeply personal. This concluding section serves as a reflection on the key takeaways and encourages readers to approach their health with newfound knowledge, confidence, and a sense of empowerment.

Recap of Key Points

Understanding Erectile Dysfunction: Revisit the fundamental aspects of erectile dysfunction, recognizing its diverse causes, the interplay of physical and psychological factors, and the impact on overall well-being.

The Science Behind Cialis: Delve into the scientific intricacies of Cialis, appreciating the role of Tadalafil, its unique mechanisms of action, and how it distinguishes itself among ED medications.

Exploring Cialis Variants: Recognize the versatility of Cialis through its daily and as-needed variants, as well as the emergence of generic options, providing individuals with choices that align with their preferences and lifestyles.

Lifestyle and Cialis: Embrace the symbiotic relationship between lifestyle choices and the effectiveness of Cialis, understanding how a holistic approach can optimize the benefits of this medication.

A Path to Spontaneity: Whether opting for the daily or as-needed variant, Cialis opens doors to spontaneity and flexibility in intimate relationships. Recognize the empowerment that comes with having a reliable ally in the journey to overcome erectile challenges. Communication and Connection: Encourage open communication between individuals and their partners, fostering understanding and shared experiences. The journey with Cialis is not just an individual one but a collaborative effort that strengthens relationships.

Continued Collaboration with Healthcare Professionals: Stress the ongoing collaboration with healthcare professionals for personalized guidance. From initial consultations to dosage adjustments, the partnership with healthcare providers is pivotal for optimal outcomes.

Ongoing Research and Development: Acknowledge the dynamic nature of medical advancements, with ongoing research and development shaping the landscape of ED treatments. Remain curious and informed about emerging innovations.

Holistic Well-being: Emphasize the importance of a holistic approach to well-being beyond ED management. The lifestyle changes and healthy habits adopted on this journey contribute to overall health and vitality. In concluding this guide, it is our hope that the information provided has illuminated the path to a healthier, more fulfilling life for those grappling with erectile dysfunction. Cialis, with its scientific foundation and diverse variants, stands as a beacon of hope in this journey. May this guide serve as a source of empowerment, enabling individuals to make informed decisions, embrace positive lifestyle changes, and approach their intimate health with confidence and resilience. Remember, the path to well-being is unique for each individual, and the choices made today pave the way for a healthier and more satisfying tomorrow.

THE END

Made in the USA
Las Vegas, NV
09 April 2024

88479529R00022